The Vibrant Dash Diet Dishes Cooking Book

Fit and Healthy Recipes to Make Incredible and Super Affordable Meals

Lola Rogers

Table of contents

Tomato Soup

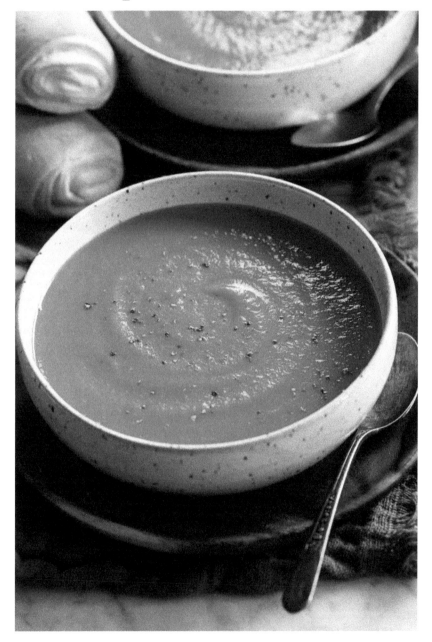

Serving: 3

Prep Time: 10 minutes

Cook Time: 6-8 hours

Ingredients:

- 4 cups water or vegetable broth
- 7 large tomatoes, ripe
- ½ cup macadamia nuts, raw
- 1 medium onion, chopped
- Sunflower seeds and pepper to taste

How To:

1. Take a nonstick skillet and add the onion.
2. Brown the onion for five minutes.
3. Add all the ingredients to a crockpot.
4. Cook for 6-8 hours on LOW.
5. Make a smooth puree by employing a blender.
6. Serve it warm and enjoy!

Nutrition (Per Serving)

Calories: 145

Fat: 12g

Carbohydrates: 8g

Protein: 6g

Pumpkin, Coconut and Sage Soup

Serving: 3

Prep Time: 10 minute

Cook Time: 30 minutes

Ingredients:

- 1 cup pumpkin, canned
- 6 cups chicken broth
- 1 cup low fat coconut almond milk
- 1 teaspoon sage, chopped
- 3 garlic cloves, peeled
- Sunflower seeds and pepper to taste

How To:

1.   Take a stockpot and add all the ingredients except coconut almond milk into it.

2.   Place stockpot over medium heat.

3.   Let it bring back a boil.

4.   Reduce heat to simmer for half-hour .

5.   Add the coconut almond milk and stir.

6.   Serve bacon and enjoy!

Nutrition (Per Serving)

Calories: 145

Fat: 12g

Carbohydrates: 8g

Protein: 6g

Classic Tuna Salad

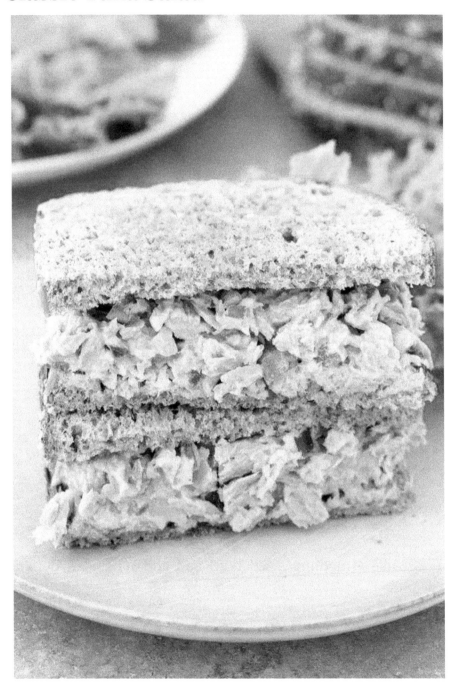

Serving: 4

Prep Time: 10 minutes

Cook Time: Nil

Ingredients:

12 ounces white tuna, in water

- ½ cup celery, diced
- 2 tablespoons fresh parsley, chopped
- 2 tablespoons low-calorie mayonnaise, low fat and low odium
- ½ teaspoon Dijon mustard
- ½ teaspoon sunflower seeds
- ¼ teaspoon fresh ground black pepper

Direction

1. Take a medium sized bowl and add tuna, parsley, and celery.

2. Mix well and add mayonnaise and mustard.

3. Season with pepper and sunflower seeds.

4.   Stir and add olives, relish, chopped pickle, onion and mix well.

5.   Serve and enjoy

Nutrition (Per Serving)

Calories: 137

Fat: 5g

Carbohydrates: 1g

Protein: 20g

Greek Salad

Serving: 4

Prep Time: 6 minutes

Cook Time: Nil

Ingredients:

- 2 cucumbers, diced
- 2 tomatoes, sliced
- 1 green lettuce, cut into thin strips
- 2 red bell peppers, cut
- ½ cup black olives pitted
- 3 ½ ounces feta cheese, cut
- 1 red onion, sliced
- 2 tablespoons olive oil
- 2 tablespoons lemon juice
- Sunflower seeds and pepper to taste

Direction

1. Dice cucumbers and slice up the tomatoes.

2.   Tear the lettuce and cut it into thin strips.

3.   De-seed and cut the peppers into strips.

4.   Take a salad bowl and mix in all the listed vegetables, add olives and feta cheese (cut into cubes).

5.   Take a small cup and mix in olive oil and lemon juice, season with sunflower seeds and pepper.

6.   Pour mixture into the salad and toss well, enjoy!

Nutrition (Per Serving)

Calories: 132

Fat: 4g

Carbohydrates: 3g

Protein: 5g

Fancy Greek Orzo Salad

Serving: 4

Prep Time: 5 minutes and 24 hours chill time

Cook Time: 10 minutes

Ingredients:

- 1 cup orzo pasta, uncooked
- ½ cup fresh parsley, minced
- 6 teaspoons olive oil
- 1 onion, chopped
- 1 ½ teaspoons oregano

How To:

1. Cook the orzo and drain them.
2. Add to a serving dish.
3. Add 2 teaspoons of oil.
4. Take another dish and add parsley, onion, remaining oil and oregano.
5. Season with sunflower seeds, pepper according to your taste.

6. Pour the mixture over the orzo and let it chill for 24 hours.

7. Serve and enjoy at lunch!

Nutrition (Per Serving)

Calories: 399

Fat: 12g

Carbohydrates: 55g

Protein:16g

Homely Tuscan Tuna Salad

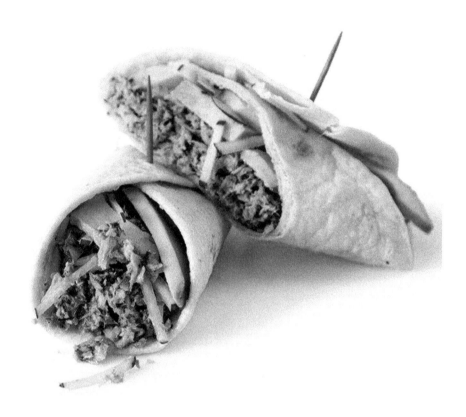

Serving: 4

Prep Time: 5-10 minutes

Cook Time: Nil

Ingredients:

- 15 ounces small white beans
- 6 ounces drained chunks of light tuna
- cherry tomatoes, quartered
- 4 scallions, trimmed and sliced
- 2 tablespoons lemon juice

How To:

Add all of the listed ingredients to a bowl and gently stir.

Season with sunflower seeds and pepper accordingly, enjoy!

Nutrition (Per Serving)

Calories: 322

Fat: 8g

Carbohydrates: 32g

Protein:30g

Asparagus Loaded Lobster Salad

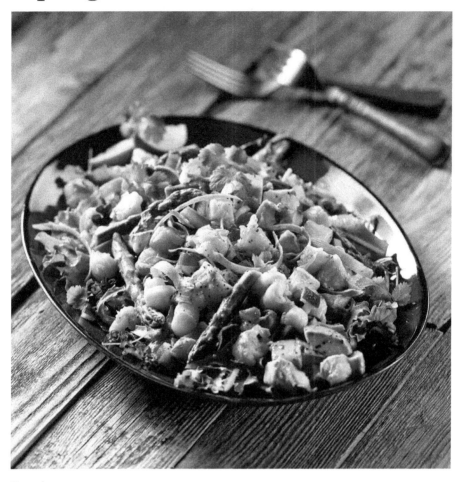

Serving: 4

Prep Time: 10 minutes

Cook Time: Nil

Ingredients:

- 8 ounces lobster, cooked and chopped
- 3 ½ cups asparagus, chopped and steamed
- 2 tablespoons lemon juice
- 4 teaspoons extra virgin olive oil
- ¼ teaspoon kosher sunflower seeds
- Pepper
- ½ cup cherry tomatoes halved
- 1 basil leaf, chopped
- 2 tablespoons red onion, diced

How To:

1.   Whisk in lemon juice, sunflower seeds, pepper in a bowl and mix with oil.

2.   Take a bowl and add the rest of the ingredients.

3.   Toss well and pour dressing on top.

Serve and enjoy!

Nutrition (Per Serving)

Calories: 247

Fat: 10g

Carbohydrates: 14g

Protein: 27g

Simple One Pot Mussels

Serving: 4

Prep Time: 10 minutes

Cook Time: 5 minutes

Ingredients:

- 2 tablespoons butter
- 2 chopped shallots
- minced garlic cloves
- ½ cup broth
- ½ cup white wine
- 2 pounds cleaned mussels
- Lemon and parsley for serving

How To:

1. Clean the mussels and take away the beard.

2. Discard any mussels that don't close when tapped against a tough surface.

3. Set your pot to Sauté mode and add chopped onion and butter.

4. Stir and sauté onions.

5. Add garlic and cook for 1 minute.

6. Add broth and wine.

7. Lock the lid and cook for five minutes on high .

8. Release the pressure naturally over 10 minutes.

9. Serve with a sprinkle of parsley and enjoy!

Nutrition (Per Serving)

Calories: 286

Fats: 14g

Carbs: 12g

Protein: 28g

Shrimp With Corn Hash

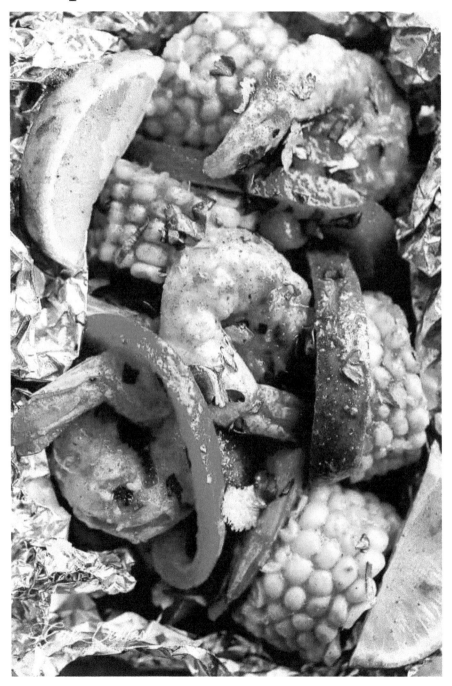

Prep time: 5 minutes

Cook time: 10 minutes

Servings: 4

Ingredients

- Olive oil – 4 tsp.
- Large shrimp - 1 pound, peeled and deveined
- Chopped red onion – ½ cup
- Red bell pepper – ½, chopped
- Fresh corn kernels – 1 ½ cup
- Halved cherry – 1 cup
- Crushed hot red pepper – ¼ tsp.
- Water – ¼ cup
- Fresh lemon juice – 1 Tbsp.
- Chopped fresh basil – 2 Tbsp.

Method

1. Heat 2 tsp. oil in a skillet.
2. Add the shrimp
3. Cook for 3 to 5 minutes. Transfer to a plate.
4. Heat remaining 2 tsp. oil in the skillet. Add bell pepper.

5. Then onion and stir-fry for 1 minute, or until softened.

6. Add tomatoes, corn, and hot pepper and cover.

7. Cook for 3 minutes.

8. Add the shrimp and reheat, stirring often, about 1 minute.

9. Stir in lemon juice and water and cook.

10. Sprinkle with basil and serve.

Nutritional Facts Per Serving

Calories: 195

Fat: 6g

Carb: 18g

Protein: 18g

Sodium 647mg

Shrimp Ceviche

Prep time: 10 minutes

Cook time: 0 minutes

Servings: 8

Ingredients

- Raw shrimp – ½ pound, cut into ¼ inch pieces
- Lemons – 2, zest and juice
- Limes -2, zest and juice
- Olive oil - 2 Tbsp.
- Cumin – 2 tsp.
- Diced red onion – ½ cup
- Diced tomato – 1 cup
- Minced garlic – 2 Tbsp.
- Black beans - 1 cup, cooked
- Diced serrano chili pepper – ¼ cup, seeds removed
- Diced cucumber – 1 cup, peeled and seeded
- Chopped cilantro – ¼ cup

Method

1.   In a bowl, place the shrimp and cover with the lemon and lime juice. Marinate for at least 3 hours.

2.   In another bowl, mix the remaining ingredients and set aside.

3.   Before serving, mix shrimp and the juice with remaining ingredients.

4.   Serve.

Nutritional Facts Per Serving

Calories: 98

Fat: 4g

Carb: 10g

Protein: 7g

Sodium 167mg

Grilled Asian Salmon

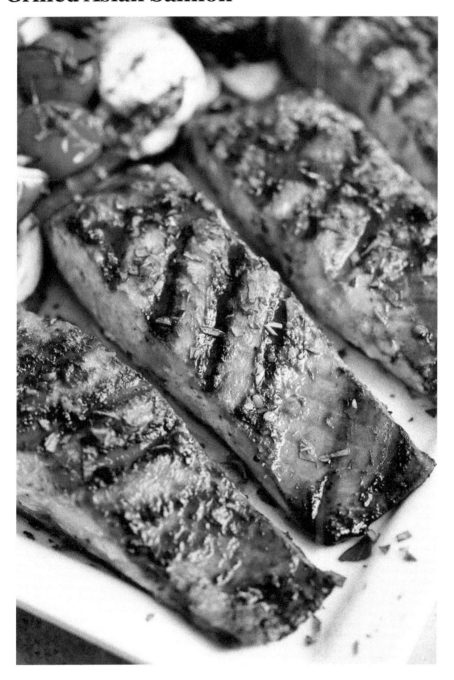

Prep time: 1 hour

Cook time: 10 minutes

Servings: 4

Ingredients

- Sesame oil – 1 Tbsp.
- Homemade soy sauce – 1 Tbsp.
- Fresh ginger – 1 Tbsp. minced
- Rice wine vinegar – 1 Tbsp.
- Salmon fillets – 4, each 4 ounces

Method

1. Combine vinegar, ginger, soy sauce, and sesame oil in a dish.

2. Add salmon and coat well. Marinate for 1 hour, turning occasionally (in the refrigerator).

3. Grease a grill and heat over medium heat.

4. Grill the salmon on 5 minutes per side or until almost opaque.

5. Serve.

Nutritional Facts Per Serving

Calories: 185

Fat: 9g

Carb: 1g

Protein: 26g

Sodium 113mg

Herb-Crusted Baked Cod

Prep time: 10 minutes

Cook time: 10 minutes

Servings: 4

Ingredients

- Herb-flavored stuffing – ¾ cup, crushed until crumbed
- Cod fillets – 4 (4 ounces each)
- Honey - ¼ cup

Method

1. Preheat the oven to 375F. Coat a baking pan with cooking spray.
2. Brush the fillets with honey. Discard the rest of the honey.
3. Place the stuffing in a bag and place a fillet in the bag.
4. Shake the bag to coat the cod well.
5. Remove the fillet and repeat with the remaining fillets.

Bake the fillets for 10 minutes or until opaque throughout.

Nutritional Facts Per Serving

Calories: 185

Fat: 1g

Carb: 23g

Protein: 21g

Sodium 163mg

Shrimp Kebabs

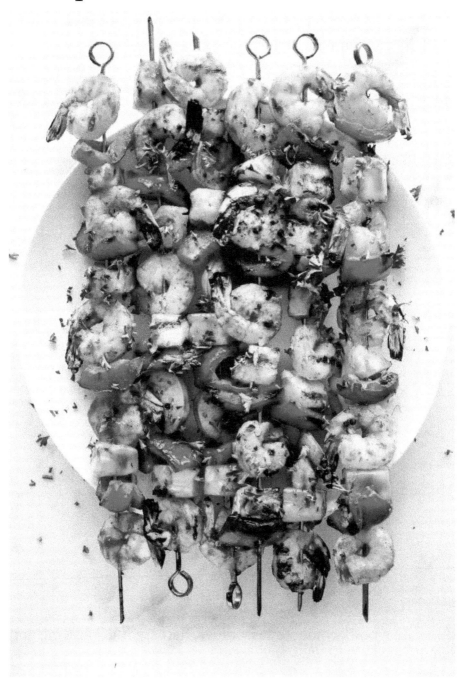

Prep time: 10 minutes

Cook time: 5 minutes

Servings: 2

Ingredients

- Lemon – 1, juiced
- Olive oil – 1 Tbsp.
- Finely minced garlic – 2 tsp.
- Finely chopped fresh tarragon – 1 tsp.
- Finely chopped fresh rosemary – 1 tsp.
- Kosher salt - ½ tsp.
- Ground black pepper – ¼ tsp.
- Shrimp – 12 pieces, peeled and deveined

Method

Soak 2 wooden skewers for 10 minutes.

1.   Preheat grill on high.

2.   In a bowl, combine seasonings, herbs, garlic, olive oil, and lemon juice.

3.   Marinade the shrimp into the lemon marinade for 5 minutes.

4.   Skewer the shrimp.

5.   Then place on the grill. Cook until shrimp is thoroughly cooked, about 2 minutes per side.

6.   Serve.

Nutritional Facts Per Serving

Calories: 105

Fat: 1g

Carb: 0g

Protein: 24g

Sodium 185mg

Roasted Salmon

Prep time: 5 minutes

Cook time: 12 minutes

Servings: 2

Ingredients

- Salmon with skin – 2 (5-ounce) pieces
- Extra-virgin olive oil – 2 tsp.
- Chopped chives – 1 Tbsp.
- Fresh tarragon leaves – 1 Tbsp.

Method

1.   Preheat the oven to 425F. Line a baking sheet with foil.

2.   Rub salmon with oil.

3.   Line a baking sheet with foil.

4.   Place salmon (skin side down).

5.   Cook for 12 minutes or until fish is cooked through. Check after 10 minutes.

6.   Serve the salmon with herbs.

Nutritional Facts Per Serving

Calories: 244

Fat: 14g

Carb: 0g

Protein: 28g

Sodium 62mg

Lamb Curry With Tomatoes And Spinach

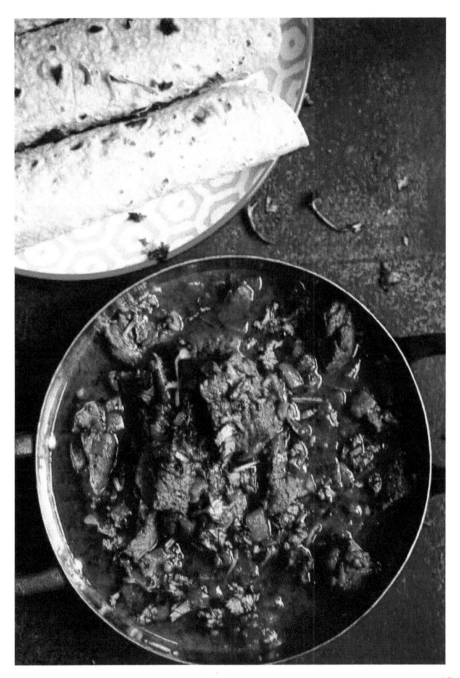

Prep time: 10 minutes

Cook time: 12 minutes

Servings: 4

Ingredients

- Olive oil – 1 tsp.
- Lean boneless lamb – 1 pound, sliced thinly
- Onion – 1, chopped
- Garlic – 3 cloves, minced
- Red bell pepper – 1, chopped
- Salt-free
- tomato paste – 2 Tbsp.
- Salt-free curry powder – 1 Tbsp.
- No-salt-added diced tomatoes – 1(15-ounce) can
- Fresh baby spinach – 10 ounces
- Low-sodium beef or vegetable broth - ½ cup
- Red wine – ¼ cup

- Chopped fresh cilantro – ¼ cup Ground black pepper to taste

Method

1.   Heat the oil in a pan.

2.   Add lamb and brown both sides, about 2 minutes.

3.   Add garlic, onion, and bell pepper. Stir-fry for 2 minutes. Stir in the curry powder and tomato paste.

4.   Add the tomatoes with juice, spinach, broth, and wine and stir to mix.

5.   Stir-fry for 3 to 4 minutes and lamb has cooked through.

6.   Remove from heat. Season with pepper and stir in cilantro.

7.   Serve.

Nutritional Facts Per Serving

Calories: 238

Fat: 7g

Carb: 14g

Protein: 27g

Sodium 167mg

Pomegranate-Marinated Leg Of Lamb

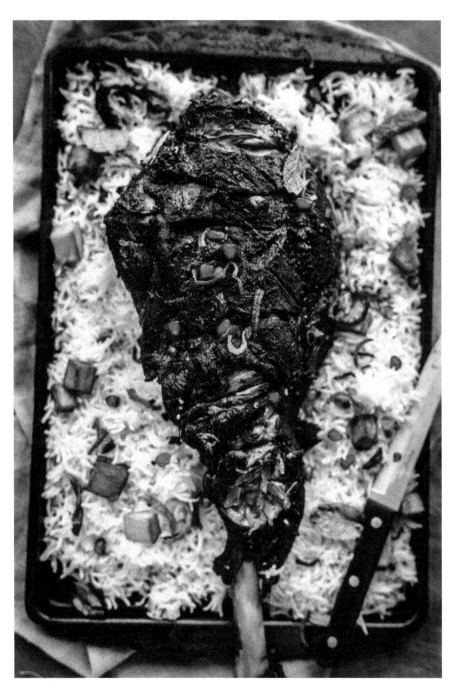

Prep time: 10 minutes

Cook time: 20 minutes

Servings: 6

Ingredients

For the marinate

- Bottled pomegranate juice - ½ cup
- Hearty red wine – ½ cup
- Ground cumin - 1 tsp.
- Dried oregano – 1 tsp.
- Crushed hot red pepper – ½ tsp.
- Garlic – 3 cloves, minced

For the lamb

- Boneless leg of lamb – 1 ¾ pound, butterflied and fat trimmed

- Kosher salt – ½ tsp.
- Olive oil spray

Method

1.   To make the marinade, whisk everything in a bowl and transfer to a zippered plastic bag.

2.   To prepare the lamb: add the lamb to the bag, press out the air, and close the bag. Marinate for 1 hour in the refrigerator.

3.   Preheat the broiler (8 inches from the source of heat).

4.   Remove the lamb from the marinade, blot with paper towels, but do not dry completely.

5.   Season with salt. Spray the broiler rack with oil.

6.   Place the lamb on the rack and broil, turning occasionally, about 20 minutes, or until lamb is browned and reaches 130F.

7.   Remove from heat, slice and serve with carving juices on top.

Nutritional Facts Per Serving

Calories: 273

Fat: 15g

Carb: 0g

Protein: 31g

Sodium 219mg

Beef Fajitas With Peppers

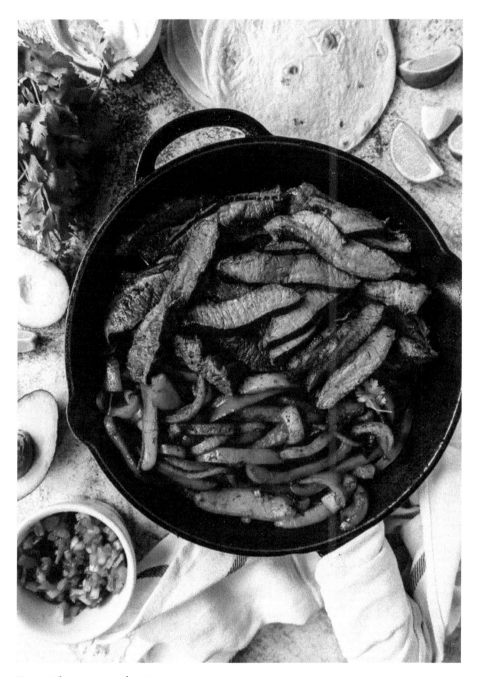

Prep time: 10 minutes

Cook time: 12 minutes

Servings: 6

Ingredients

- Olive oil – 2 tsp. plus more for the spray
- Sirloin steak – 1 pound, cut into bite-size pieces
- Red bell pepper – 1, chopped
- Green bell pepper – 1, chopped
- Red onion – 1, chopped
- Garlic - 2 cloves, minced
- DASH friendly Mexican seasoning – 1 Tbsp. (or any seasoning without salt)
- Boston lettuce leaves – 12 for serving
- Lime wedges or corn tortillas for serving

Method

Heat oil in a skillet.

Add half of the sirloin and cook until browned on both sides, about 2 minutes. Transfer to a plate.

Then repeat with the remaining sirloin.

Heat the 2 tsp. oil in the skillet.

Add onion, bell peppers, and garlic, cook and stir for 7 minutes or until tender.

Stir in the beef with any juices and the seasoning. Transfer to a plate.

Fill lettuce lead with beef mixture and drizzle lime juice on top.

Roll up and serve.

Nutritional Facts Per Serving

Calories: 231

Fat: 12g

Carb: 6g

Protein: 24g

Sodium 59mg

Pork Medallions With Herbs De Provence

Prep time: 5 minutes

Cook time: 10 minutes

Servings: 2

Ingredients

- Pork tenderloin – 8 ounces, cut into 6 pieces (crosswise)
- Ground black pepper to taste
- Herbs de Provence – ½ tsp.
- Dry white wine – ¼ cup

Method

1. Season the pork with black pepper.
2. Place the pork between waxed paper sheets and roll with a rolling pin until about ¼ inch thick.
3. Cook the pork in a pan for 2 to 3 minutes on each side.
4. Remove from heat and season with the herb.
5. Place the pork on plates and keep warm.
6. Cook the wine in the pan until boiling. Scrape to get the brown bits from the bottom.

7. Serve pork with the sauce.

Nutritional Facts Per Serving

Calories: 120

Fat: 2g

Carb: 1g

Protein: 24g

Sodium 62mg

Baked Chicken

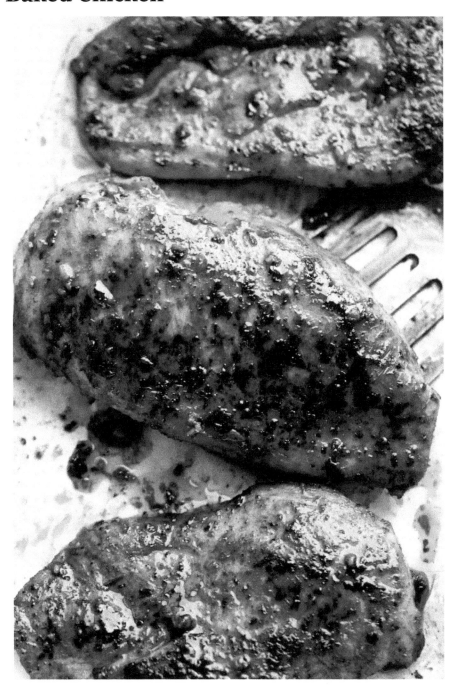

Prep time: 10 minutes

Cook time: 1 hour

Servings: 4

Ingredients

- Chicken – 3 to 4 pound, cut into parts
- Olive oil – 3 Tbsp.
- Thyme – ½ tsp.
- Sea salt – ¼ tsp.
- Ground black pepper
- Low-sodium chicken stock – ½ cup

Method

1. Preheat the oven to 400F.
2. Rub oil over chicken pieces. Sprinkle with salt, thyme, and pepper.
3. Place chicken in the roasting pan.
4. Bake in the oven for 30 minutes.
5. Then lower the heat to 350F.
6. Bake for 15 to 30 minutes more or until juice runs clear.
7. Serve.

Nutritional Facts Per Serving

Calories: 550

Fat: 19g

Carb: 0g

Protein: 91g

Sodium 480mg

The Mean Green Smoothie

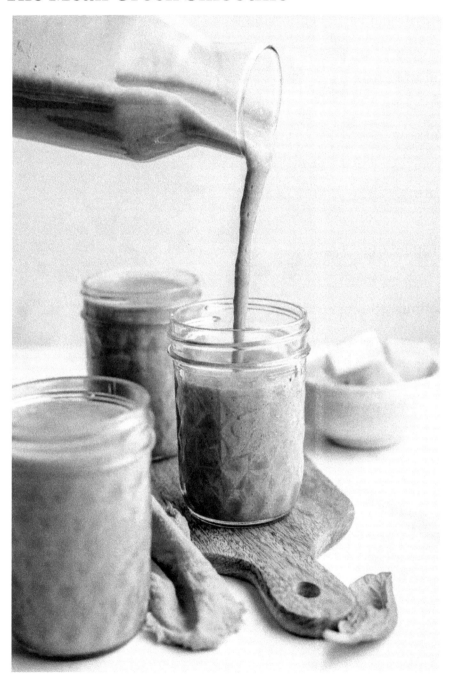

Serving: 2

Prep Time: 5 minutes

Ingredients:

- 1 avocado
- 1 handful spinach, chopped
- Cucumber, 2 inch slices, peeled
- 1 lime, chopped
- Handful of grapes, chopped
- 5 dates, stoned and chopped
- 1 cup apple juice (fresh)

How To:

1. Add all the listed ingredients to your blender.
2. Blend until smooth.
3. Add a few ice cubes and serve the smoothie.
4. Enjoy!

Nutrition (Per Serving)

Calories: 200

Fat: 10g

Carbohydrates: 14g

Protein 2g

Mint Flavored Pear Smoothie

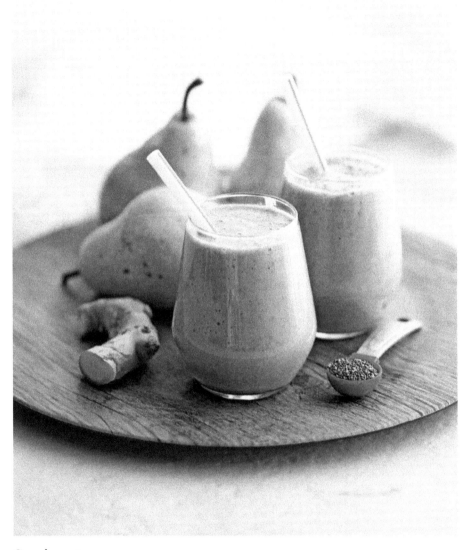

Serving: 2

Prep Time: 5 minutes

Ingredients:

- ¼ honey dew
- 2 green pears, ripe
- ½ apple, juiced 1 cup ice cubes
- ½ cup fresh mint leaves

How To:

Add the listed ingredients to your blender and blend until smooth. Serve chilled!

Nutrition (Per Serving)

Calories: 200

Fat: 10gCarbohydrates: 14g

Protein 2g

Chilled Watermelon Smoothie

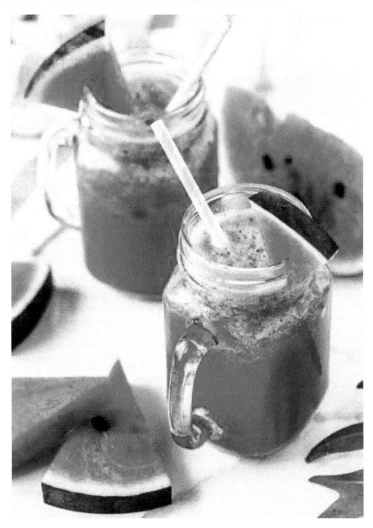

Serving: 2

Prep Time: 5 minutes

Ingredients:

- 1 cup watermelon chunks
- ½ cup coconut water
- 1 ½ teaspoons lime juice
- 4 mint leaves
- 4 ice cubes

How To:

1.   Add the listed ingredients to your blender and blend until smooth.
2.   Serve chilled! Nutrition (Per Serving)

Calories: 200

Fat: 10g

Carbohydrates: 14g

Protein 2g

Banana Ginger Medley

Serving: 2

Prep Time: 5 minutes

Ingredients:

- 1 banana, sliced
- ¾ cup vanilla yogurt
- 1 tablespoon honey
- ½ teaspoon ginger, grated

How To:

1.   Add the listed ingredients to your blender and blend until smooth.
2.   Serve chilled!

Nutrition (Per Serving)

Calories: 200

Fat: 10g

Carbohydrates: 14g

Protein 2g

Banana and Almond Flax Glass

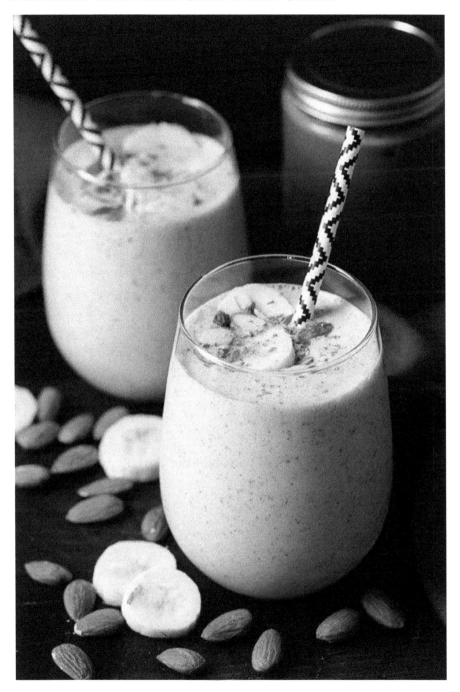

Serving: 2

Prep Time: 5 minutes

Ingredients:

- 1 ripe frozen banana, diced
- 2/3 cup unsweetened almond milk
- 1/3 cup fat free plain Greek Yogurt
- 1 ½ tablespoons almond butter
- 1 tablespoon flaxseed meal
- 1 teaspoon honey
- 2-3 drops almond extract

How To:

Add the listed ingredients to your blender and blend until smooth
Serve chilled!

Nutrition (Per Serving)

Calories: 200

Fat: 10g

Carbohydrates: 14g

Protein 2g

Satisfying Honey and Coconut Porridge

Serving: 8

Prep Time: 10 minutes

Cook Time: 8 hours

Ingredients:

- 4 cups light coconut milk
- 3 cups apple juice
- 2 ¼ cups coconut flour
- 1 teaspoon ground cinnamon
- ¼ cup honey

How To:

1. In a Slow Cooker, add the coconut milk, apple juice, flour, cinnamon and honey.
2. Stir well.
3. Close lid and cook on LOW for 8 hours.
4. Open lid and stir.
5. Serve with an additional seasoning of fresh fruits.

6.   Enjoy!

Nutrition (Per Serving)

Calories: 372

Fat: 14g

Carbohydrates: 56g

Protein: 8g

Pure Maple Glazed Carrots

Serving: 6

Prep Time: 10 minutes

Cook Time: 8 hours

Ingredients:

- ¼ cup pure maple syrup
- ½ teaspoon ground ginger
- ¼ teaspoon ground nutmeg
- ½ teaspoon salt
- Juice of 1 orange
- 1-pound baby carrots

How To:

1. Take a small bowl and whisk in syrup, nutmeg, ginger, salt, orange juice.

2. Add carrots to your Slow Cooker and pour the maple syrup.

3. Toss to coat.

4. Close lid and cook on LOW for 8 hours.

5.   Serve and enjoy!

Nutrition (Per Serving)

Calories: 76

Fat: 1g

Carbohydrates: 19g

Protein: 76g

Ginger and Orange "Beets"

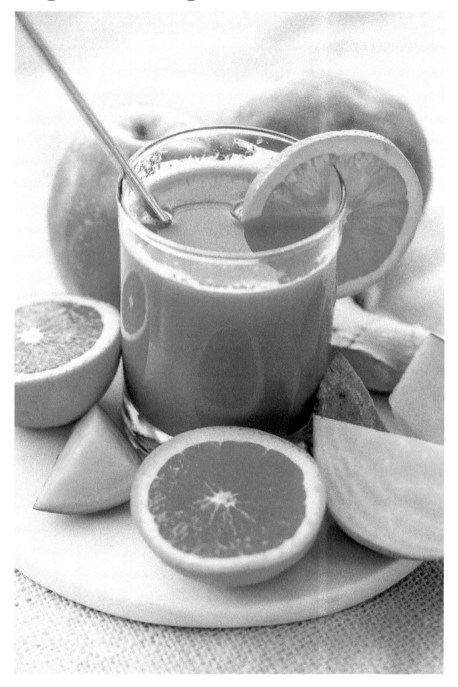

Serving: 6

Prep Time: 20 minutes

Cook Time: 8 hours

Ingredients:

- 2 pounds beets, peeled and cut into wedges
- Juice of 2 oranges
- Zest of 1 orange
- 1 teaspoon fresh ginger, grated
- 1 tablespoon honey
- 1 tablespoon apple cider vinegar
- 1/8 teaspoon fresh ground black pepper
- Sea salt

How To:

1.   Add beets, zest, orange juice, ginger, honey, pepper, salt and vinegar to your Slow Cooker.

2.   Stir well.

3.   Close lid and cook on LOW for 8 hours.

4.   Serve and enjoy!

Nutrition (Per Serving)

Calories: 108

Fat: 1g

Carbohydrates: 25g

Protein: 3g

Pineapple Rice

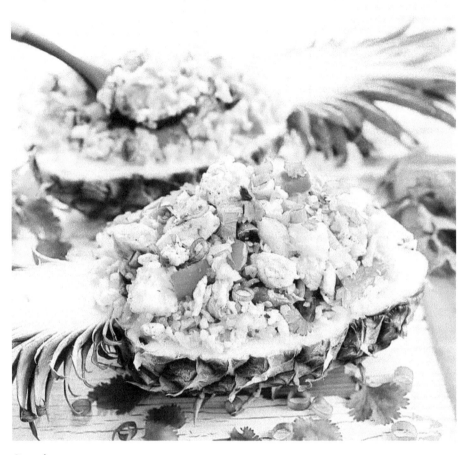

Serving: 2

Prep Time: 10 minutes

Cook Time: 2 hours

Ingredients:

- 1 cup rice

- 2 cups water

- 1 small cauliflower, florets separated and chopped

- ½ small pineapple, peeled and chopped

- Salt and pepper as needed

- 1 teaspoon olive oil

How To:

1.   Add rice, cauliflower, pineapple, water, oil, salt and pepper to your Slow Cooker.

2.   Gently stir.

3.   Place lid and cook on HIGH for 2 hours.

4.   Fluff the rice with fork and season with more salt and pepper if needed.

5.   Divide between serving platters and enjoy!

Nutrition (Per Serving)

Calories: 152

Fat: 4g

Carbohydrates: 18g

Protein: 4g

Creative Lemon and Broccoli Dish

Serving: 6

Prep Time: 10 minutes

Cook Time: 15 minutes

Ingredients:

- 2 heads broccocli, separated into florets
- 2 teaspoons extra virgin olive oil
- 1 teaspoon sunflower seeds
- ½ teaspoon black pepper
- 1 garlic clove, minced
- ½ teaspoon lemon juice

How To:

1.   Pre-heat your oven to 400 degrees F.

2.   Take a large sized bowl and add broccoli florets.

3.   Drizzle olive oil and season with pepper, sunflower seeds and garlic.

4.   Spread broccoli out in a single even layer on a baking sheet.

5.   Bake for 15-20 minutes until fork tender.

6.   Squeeze lemon juice on top.

7. Serve and enjoy!

Nutrition (Per Serving)

Calories: 49

Fat: 1.9g

Carbohydrates: 7g

Protein: 3g

Zingy Onion and Thyme Crackers

Serving: 75 crackers

Prep Time: 15 minutes

Cooking Time: 120 minutes

Ingredients:

- 1 garlic clove, minced
- 1 cup sweet onion, coarsely chopped
- 2 teaspoons fresh thyme leaves
- ¼ cup avocado oil
- ¼ teaspoon garlic powder
- Freshly ground black pepper
- ¼ cup sunflower seeds
- 1 ½ cups roughly ground flax seeds

How To:

1.   Preheat your oven to 225 degrees F.

2.   Line two baking sheets with parchment paper and keep it on the side.

3.   Add garlic, onion, thyme, oil, sunflower seeds, and pepper to a kitchen appliance .

4.   Add sunflower and flax seeds, pulse until pureed.

5.   Transfer the batter to prepared baking sheets and spread evenly, dig crackers

6.   Bake for hour .

7.   Remove parchment paper and flip crackers, bake for an additional hour.

8.   If crackers are thick, it'll take longer .

9.   Remove from oven and allow them to cool.

10.   Enjoy!

Nutrition (Per Serving)

Total Carbs: 0.8g

Fiber: 0.2g

Protein: 0.4g

Fat: 2.7g

Crunchy Flax and Almond Crackers

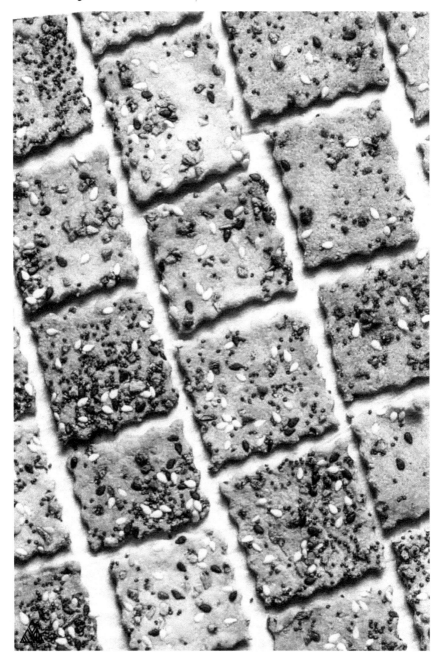

Serving: 20-24 crackers

Prep Time: 15 minutes

Cooking Time: 60 minutes

Ingredients:

- ½ cup ground flaxseeds
- ½ cup almond flour
- 1 tablespoon coconut flour
- 2 tablespoons shelled hemp seeds
- ¼ teaspoon sunflower seeds
- 1 egg white
- 2 tablespoons unsalted almond butter, melted

How To:

1.   Preheat your oven to 300 degrees F.

2.   Line a baking sheet with parchment paper, keep it on the side.

3.   Add flax, almond, coconut flour, hemp seed, seeds to a bowl and blend .

4.   Add albumen and melted almond butter, mix until combined.

5.   Transfer dough to a sheet of parchment paper and canopy with another sheet of paper.

6.   Roll out dough.

7.   dig crackers and bake for hour .

8.   allow them to cool and enjoy!

Nutrition (Per Serving)

Total Carbs: 1.2

Fiber: 1g

Protein: 2g

Fat: 6g

Basil and Tomato Baked Eggs

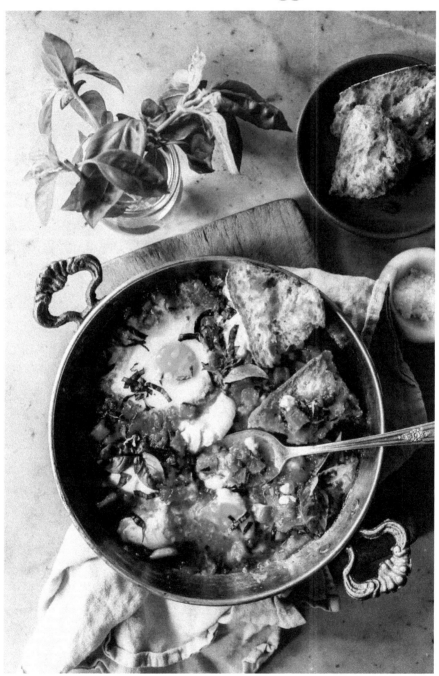

Serving: 2

Prep Time: 10 minutes

Cook Time: 15 minutes

Ingredients:

- 1/2 garlic clove, minced
- 1/2 cup canned tomatoes
- ¼ cup fresh basil leaves, roughly chopped
- 1/4 teaspoon chili powder
- 1/2 tablespoon olive oil
- 2 whole eggs
- Pepper to taste

How To:

1. Preheat your oven to 375 degrees F.

2. Take alittle baking dish and grease with vegetable oil .

3. Add garlic, basil, tomatoes chili, vegetable oil into a dish and stir.

4. Crack eggs into a dish, keeping space between the 2 .

5. Sprinkle the entire dish with sunflower seeds and pepper.

6.   Place in oven and cook for 12 minutes until eggs are set and tomatoes are bubbling.

7.   Serve with basil on top.

Enjoy!

Nutrition (Per Serving)

Calories: 235

Fat: 16g

Carbohydrates: 7g

Protein: 14g

Cool Mushroom Munchies

Serving: 2

Prep Time: 5 minute

Cook Time: 10 minutes

Ingredients:

- 4 Portobello mushroom caps
- 3 tablespoons coconut aminos
- 2 tablespoons sesame oil
- 1 tablespoon fresh ginger, minced
- 1 small garlic clove, minced

How To:

1. Set your broiler to low, keeping the rack 6 inches from the heating source.

2. Wash mushrooms under cold water and transfer them to a baking sheet (top side down).

3. Take a bowl and blend in vegetable oil , garlic, coconut aminos, ginger and pour the mixture over the mushrooms tops .

4. Cook for 10 minutes.

5.   Serve and enjoy!

Nutrition (Per Serving)

Calories: 196

Fat: 14g

Carbohydrates: 14g

Protein: 7g

Banana and Buckwheat Porridge

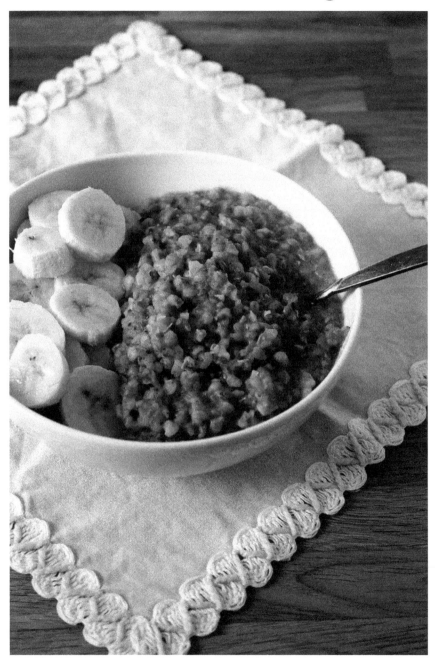

Serving: 2

Prep Time: 10 minutes

Cook Time: 15 minutes

Ingredients:

- 1 cup of water
- 1 cup buckwheat groats
- 2 big grapefruits, peeled and sliced
- 1 tablespoon ground cinnamon
- 3-4 cups almond milk
- 2 tablespoons natural almond butter

How To:

1. Take a medium-sized saucepan and add buckwheat and water.

2. Place the pan over medium heat and convey to a boil.

3. Keep cooking until the buckwheat absorbs the water.

4. Reduce heat to low and add almond milk, stir gently.

5. Add the remainder of the ingredients (except the grapefruits).

6. Stir and take away from the warmth .

7. Transfer into cereal bowls and add grapefruit chunks.

8.   Serve and enjoy!

Nutrition (Per Serving)

Calories: 223

Fat: 4g

Carbohydrates: 4g

Protein: 7g

Wedge Salad Skewers

Ingredients

- One head of iceberg lettuce (cut into wedge pieces)
- Four Roma tomatoes cut in half
- One red onion (cut into 1-inch pieces)
- Two avocados cut into 1-inch pieces
- Five slices of bacon cooked and cut into thirds
- One cucumber (sliced (peeled or unpeeled))
- Eight wooden skewers
- Two green onions (diced)
- 1 5 oz container blue cheese crumbles
- One bottle blue cheese dressing

Instructions

1.   One skewer at a time adds an iceberg wedge, tomato, onion, avocado, two pieces of bacon, every other iceberg wedge, and then cucumber.

2.   Continue till all skewers have been made, then garnish with crumbled blue cheese, blue cheese dressing, and diced leafy green onions.

Nutrition

Calories: 238kcal, Fat: 19g, Saturated fat: 6gCholesterol: 25mg Sodium:

401mgPotassium: 573mgCarbohydrates: 10gFiber: 5g Sugar: 3gProtein:

8gVitamin A: 890%Vitamin C: 13.9%Calcium: 144%Iron: 0.9%

Low Sodium Sheet Pan Chicken Fajitas

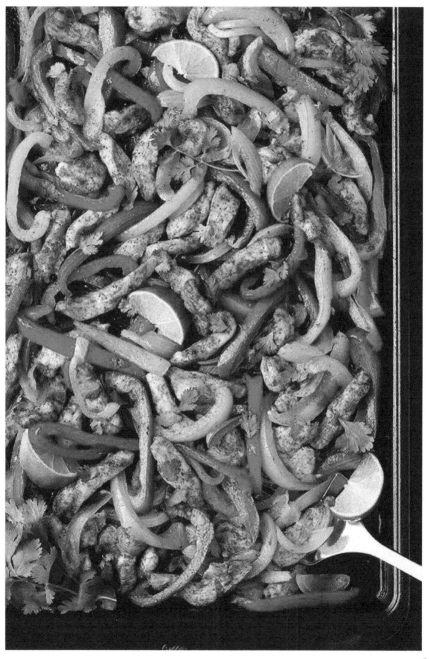

Ingredients

- Two lbs chicken breast tenderloin each sliced in half lengthwise
- One green pepper sliced
- One red bell pepper sliced
- One Vidalia onion sliced
- Olive oil spray
- One tablespoon olive oil Seasoning:
- One teaspoon chili powder
- 1/2 teaspoon smoked paprika
- 1/2 teaspoon garlic powder
- 1/2 teaspoon onion powder 1/2
- teaspoon dried oregano
- 1/2 teaspoon dried cilantro
- 1/2 teaspoon cumin
- 1/4 teaspoon cayenne pepper

Instructions

1. Preheat oven to 350 degrees F.

2. Apply a coat on a sheet pan with vegetable oil spray.

3. Spread pepper and onion slices onto a prepared sheet pan.

4. Place chicken slices on top of vegetables.

5.   Combine seasoning ingredients and stir to mix .

6.   Drizzle seasoning mixture over chicken, peppers, and onion.

7.   Sprinkle 1 tbsp of vegetable oil over chicken, peppers, and onion.

8.   Gently toss ingredients to distribute seasoning and oil evenly. (make sure chicken strips aren't overlapping)

9.   Bake for 20 min or until chicken reaches 165 deg F.

10.   Serve in warm low sodium tortillas.

11.   Top together with your favorite toppings! i really like cheddar and soured cream .

Nutrition Facts

Calories 168Calories from Fat 36 Fat 4g6% Sodium 140mg6% Potassium 531mg15% Carbohydrates 5g2% Fiber 1g4% Sugar 3g3% Protein 24g48%

Vitamin C 34.3mg42% Calcium 17mg2% Iron 0.8mg4%

Pineapple Protein Smoothie

Ingredients

- 3/4 cup milk
- 3/4 cup pineapple chunks
- 1/2 cup ice
- 3/4 cup canned chickpeas (rinsed and drained)
- 2 tbsp almond butter
- Two pitted dates
- 2 tsp ground turmeric

Directions

Blend all ingredients until smooth.

Nutrients Calories: 461

Spinach Sunshine Smoothie Bowl

Ingredients

- One packed cup baby spinach
- One banana
- 1 cup of orange juice
- 1/2 avocado
- 1/2 cup ice cubes
- Blueberries (optional)
- Diced pineapple (optional)
- Ground flaxseeds (optional)

Directions

Process the spinach, banana, fruit juice , avocado, and ice during a blender until very smooth.

Serve topped with blueberries, diced pineapple, and ground flaxseeds.

Almond Butter Berry Smoothie

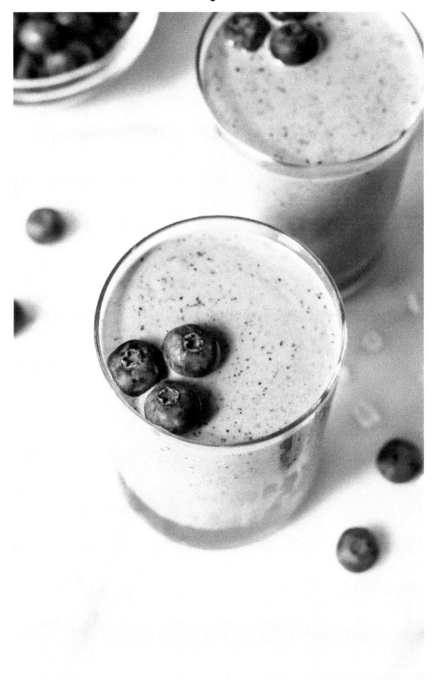

Ingredients

- 1/4 cup 1% low-fat milk
- 1/2 medium ripe banana
- 1 tbsp creamy almond butter
- 1 cup fresh or frozen raspberries
- 1/2 cup crushed ice

Directions

Blend all ingredients until smooth and enjoy!

Extreme Balsamic Chicken

Serving: 4

Prep Time: 10 minutes

Cook Time: 35 minutes

Ingredients:

- 3 boneless chicken breasts, skinless
- Sunflower seeds to taste
- ¼ cup almond flour
- 2/3 cups low-fat chicken broth
- 1 ½ teaspoons arrowroot
- ½ cup low sugar raspberry preserve
- 1 ½ tablespoons balsamic vinegar

How To:

1.   Cut pigeon breast into bite-sized pieces and season them with seeds.

2.   Dredge the chicken pieces in flour and shake off any excess.

3.   Take a non-stick skillet and place it over medium heat.

4.   Add chicken to the skillet and cook for quarter-hour , ensuring to show them half-way through.

5.   Remove chicken and transfer to platter.

6.   Add arrowroot, broth, raspberry preserve to the skillet and stir.

7.   Stir in balsamic vinegar and reduce heat to low, stir-cook for a couple of minutes.

8.   Transfer the chicken back to the sauce and cook for quarter-hour more.

9.   Serve and enjoy!

Nutrition (Per Serving)

Calories: 546

Fat: 35g

Carbohydrates: 11g

Protein: 44g

Tomato and Cheese Wrap

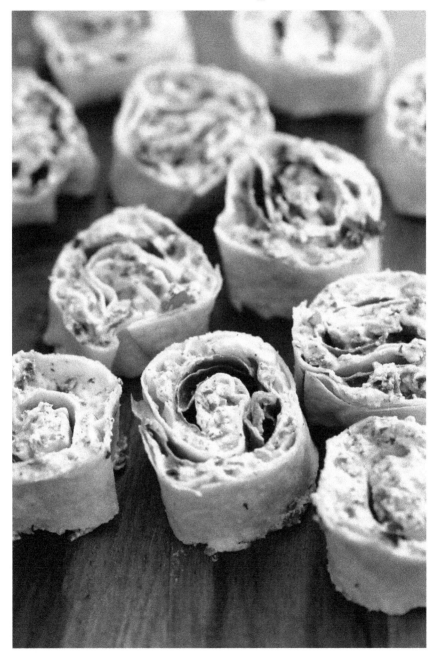

Ingredients

- Tortillas-2 tortilla -92 grams

- mayonnaise-like dressing-Regular, with salt-2 tbsp-29.4 grams

- Tomatoes-Two medium whole -246 grams

- Lettuce-2 cup shredded-144 grams

- Cheddar cheese-2 oz-56.7 grams

Directions

1. Lightly spread mayo on tortilla shell.

2. Cut tomatoes however you like them.

3. Layer ingredients, spreading them over the tortilla.

4. Tuck up about an inch the side of the shell you've decided is the bottom and roll up the wrap. Enjoy!

Nutrition

Calories638Carbs66gFat32gProtein25gFiber7gNet carbs59gSodium1236mgCholesterol63mg

Peanut butter yogurt

Ingredients

- Nonfat greek yogurt-1 cup-240 grams
- Peanut butter-2 tbsp-32 grams
- Vanilla extract-1 tsp-2.2 grams

Directions

Combine ingredients and enjoy it!

Nutrition

Calories345Carbs16gFat17gProtein32gFiber2gNet

carbs15gSodium223mgCholesterol12mg

Peanut Butter & Carrots

Ingredients

- Peanut butter-4 tbsp-64 grams
- Carrots-2 cup chopped-256 grams

Directions

Spread peanut butter on carrots and enjoy!

Nutrition

Calories482Carbs38gFat33gProtein18gFiber12gNet

carbs26gSodium188mgCholesterol0mg

Cucumber Tomato Salad with Tuna

Ingredients

- Tomatoes-Two medium whole -246 grams
- Lettuce-1 cup shredded-36 grams
- Cucumber-With peel, raw-One cucumber-301 grams
- Tuna-One can-165 grams

Directions

1. Chop vegetables and lettuce.
2. Toss together with the tuna and enjoy it!

Nutrition

Calories237Carbs22gFat2gProtein37gFiber5gNet

carbs17gSodium436mgCholesterol59mg

Peanut butter and Jelly

Ingredients

- Multi-grain bread-Four slices regular-104 grams
- Butter-Unsalted-2 tsp-9.5 grams
- Peanut butter-Smooth style, without salt-3 tbsp-48 grams
- Jams and preserves-2 tbsp-40 grams

Directions

1.   Toast the bread, and it's optionally. Drizzle1/2 teaspoon of butter on all sides of the bread.

2.   Spread butter on one side and jam on another side.

Nutrition

Calories742Carbs83gFat37gProtein25gFiber11gNet

carbs73gSodium418mgCholesterol20mg

Chicken Scampi Pasta

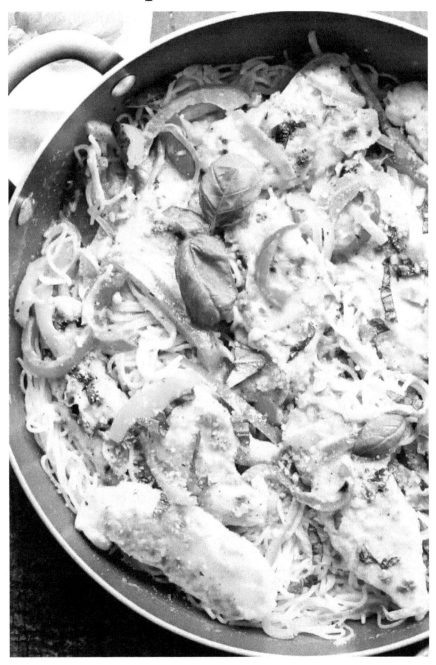

Ingredients

- 1 pound of thinly-sliced chicken cutlets, cut into 1/2-inch-thick strips

- Three tablespoons olive oil

- Eight tablespoons unsalted butter, cubed

- Six cloves garlic, sliced

- 1/2 teaspoon crushed red pepper flakes

- 1/2 cup dry white wine

- 12 ounces angel hair pasta

- One teaspoon lemon zest plus the juice of 1 large lemon

- 1/2 cup freshly grated Parmesan

- 1/2 cup chopped fresh Italian parsley

Directions

1.   Take a huge pot of salted water to a boil for the pasta. Sprinkle the chook with a couple of salts. Heat a huge skillet over medium-high warmth until hot, then upload the oil. Working in 2 batches, brown the chook until golden however not cooked through, 2 to a couple of minutes keep with batch. Remove the chicken to a plate.

2.   Melt four tablespoons of the butter within the skillet. Add the garlic and crimson pepper flakes and cook dinner until the garlic begins to show golden at the sides , 30 seconds to 1 minute. Add the wine, deliver to a simmer, and cook dinner till reduced by using half, approximately 2 minutes. Remove from the heat .

3.   Meanwhile, cook dinner the pasta till very hard , reserving 1 cup of the pasta water. Add the pasta and 3/four cup pasta water to the skillet alongside the hen, lemon peel and juice, and therefore the last four tablespoons butter. Return the skillet to medium-low warmness and gently stir the pasta until the butter is melted, including the last word 1/four pasta water if the pasta appears too dry. Remove the skillet from the heat, sprinkle with the cheese and parsley and toss before serving.

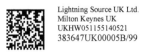